CUPPING THERAPY FOR CELLULITE

A Complete Guide On Unveiling The Art To Smooth Skin And Cupping Odyssey To Wellness

WALTER ZYAIRE

No part of this book may be reproduced, stored in a retrieval system, or transmitted in any form or by any means, electronic, mechanical, photocopying, recording, or otherwise, without the express written permission of the author, with the exception of small extracts in critical reviews or articles.

DISCLAIMER

The information in this book is intended only for general informational purposes; it should not be used in lieu of professional advice or medical care. Since the author is not licensed to practice therapy, the information offered should not be used in place of the expertise, judgment, or guidance of qualified mental health or medical professionals. Readers are encouraged to consult therapists, medical specialists, or other qualified authorities regarding their particular situation and needs. The publisher and author disclaim all liability for any actions or decisions taken by readers based on the information in this book. Results may vary from person to person and this book's approaches, procedures, and strategies may not be suitable in all circumstances. Considering unique situations and consulting a qualified expert are essential when choosing the right course of action. Neither the publisher nor the author recommend or guarantee the efficacy of any therapy or treatment that is indicated in this book. Because the information is

TABLE OF CONTENTS

ABOUT THE BOOK

The book "Cupping Therapy for Cellulite" provides practitioners and those looking for efficient ways to reduce cellulite with cupping therapy with a thorough how-to manual. The book's goal and welcome are presented in the introduction, which also establishes the significance of cupping therapy in treating cellulite-related issues.

Building a thorough grasp of cellulite—including its description, origins, and effects on body image—is the main goal of the first few chapters. By clearing up common misconceptions, readers are prepared to investigate cupping therapy as a potential cellulite reduction alternative with a foundation of knowledge.

The following sections explore the fundamentals of cupping therapy, including its origins, history, and different procedures. Comprehensive research findings, expert perspectives, and an analysis of the mechanisms via which cupping targets cellulite are included in this detailed exploration of the science behind cupping for cellulite.

After that, readers are taken through a variety of cupping procedures designed expressly to reduce cellulite, including massage, flash, silicone, wet, and dry cupping. A separate chapter discusses choosing the right equipment and cups, with a focus on safety measures to guarantee a successful and risk-free session.

Step-by-step instructions, post-cupping care, and session preparation are just a few of the practical components of cupping therapy that are described in detail. To provide a comprehensive approach for better outcomes, the book also examines the synergy between cupping therapy and other wellness activities, such as food, exercise, skincare routines, and other therapies.

Before-and-after pictures and real-life success stories give readers concrete proof of the effectiveness of cupping therapy for cellulite. The book covers typical problems and offers workable answers, making sure both practitioners and clients are prepared to face any roadblocks.

The book takes a look at the future of cupping therapy, examining current studies, breakthroughs, and new developments in the industry. Incorporating cupping into common wellness treatments, the book highlights its applicability in the changing field of cellulite reduction and overall health.

CHAPTER ONE

OVERVIEW OF CUPPING THERAPY FOR CELLULITE

CONCERNING CUPPING THERAPY

The ancient healing technique known as cupping therapy, which has roots in many different cultures, has gained more attention in the wellness community these days. Using cups applied to the skin, this therapeutic method encourages blood flow, supports the body's natural healing processes, and creates suction. Although its origins are said to be in traditional Chinese medicine, cupping therapy has also been used in various parts of the world, including the Middle East and Europe, demonstrating the diversity of its cultural past.

Using cups to apply pressure to particular body parts, usually made of silicone, glass, or bamboo, is the practice of cupping treatment. There are several ways to work with the cups: you can use them for dynamic cupping, which involves moving them over the skin, or stationary cupping, which involves leaving them in one spot. The suction that the cups create is believed to encourage the balance of Yin and Yang, which are essential ideas in traditional Chinese medicine, and to encourage the movement of Qi, or life force, within the body.

THE RELATIONSHIP BETWEEN CELLULITE AND CUPPING

A fascinating feature of cupping therapy is its link to treating cellulite, a common cosmetic issue that primarily affects women. Skin that has dimples, which are frequently seen on the thighs, buttocks, and abdomen, is a sign of cellulite.

Cellulite can affect a person's self-esteem and body image even though it is not a medical disease. The idea behind the relationship between cupping therapy and cellulite reduction is that the suction generated by the cups aids in the breakdown of fat deposits and enhances blood flow in the desired regions.

There is more to cupping therapy than just physical manipulation when it comes to reducing cellulite. Cupping proponents assert that the procedure also facilitates lymphatic drainage, which helps get rid of extra fluid and toxins that make cellulite form. Furthermore, it's believed that better blood circulation will deliver more nutrients and oxygen to the treated regions, enhancing the general health and suppleness of the skin.

It is important to approach cupping with a nuanced attitude, just as with any other alternative medicine. Many personal accounts and anecdotal evidence support the effectiveness of cupping therapy for cellulite removal, but there isn't much scientific research on the subject. However, cupping has a long history in many different cultures, and its continued use in contemporary wellness circles attests to its enduring allure and mystery.

CHAPTER TWO
KNOWING ABOUT CELLULITE
MEANING AND REASONS

Cellulite is a prevalent aesthetic issue that impacts the skin's look, especially in regions like the thighs, buttocks, and abdomen where there are underlying fat deposits. It is distinguished by a lumpy or dimpled look that frequently resembles an orange peel. Cellulite is regarded as a cosmetic concern rather than a medical disease despite being quite common.

Although the precise etiology of cellulite is unknown, several factors, including heredity, hormonal fluctuations, and lifestyle choices are thought to be involved.

Cellulite is largely influenced by genetics since specific genetic factors can affect the distribution and structure of fat under the skin. Cellulite production can also result from hormonal changes, particularly during adolescence, pregnancy, and menopause. Hormones like progesterone and estrogen are involved in controlling blood flow and fat storage, which impacts the appearance of cellulite. Furthermore, a sedentary way of living, unhealthful eating habits, and dehydration are lifestyle variables that might cause or exacerbate cellulite.

CELLULITE'S EFFECT ON BODY IMAGE

One complicated and individualized component of this cosmetic concern is the effect of cellulite on body image. The emergence of cellulite on the body can cause feelings of self-consciousness and low confidence in many people. The unfavorable image of cellulite is frequently influenced by societal beauty standards, which create unreasonable expectations that can further damage a person's self-esteem. The media's presentation of immaculate skin and unattainable body ideals can increase the pressure on persons with cellulite to meet these standards, which can have a serious psychological impact.

One of the most prevalent myths about cellulite is that it may only be caused by being overweight or leading an unhealthy lifestyle. Although cellulite can be less noticeable in people who follow a healthy weight and lifestyle, it is not limited to those who have too much body fat. Genetic and hormonal factors can cause cellulite in people who lead active lives and maintain a healthy body weight.

The idea that cellulite is a condition that exclusively affects women is another fallacy. Cellulite can affect men as well, albeit it is less common in men because of variations in skin structure and fat distribution.

Cellulite is a complex cosmetic issue impacted by a mix of lifestyle, hormonal, and genetic variables. It can have a substantial effect on body image, frequently resulting in low confidence and feelings of self-consciousness. It's important to dispel myths regarding cellulite because it affects people of all genders and body shapes and isn't just a result of being overweight or leading a bad lifestyle. Comprehending the intricacies of cellulite helps cultivate a pragmatic and empathetic outlook, thereby endorsing body positivity and self-acceptance.

CHAPTER THREE

FUNDAMENTALS OF CUPPING THERAPY

THE ORIGINS AND HISTORY OF CUPPING

The origins of cupping therapy, a traditional form of healing, date back thousands of years. Its roots can be traced back to several antiquated societies, including Egyptian, Chinese, and Middle Eastern traditions. Cupping was first known to be used as a therapeutic technique to treat a variety of illnesses in ancient Egypt. Cupping has been used in traditional Chinese medicine for more than 2,000 years, to balance the body's "qi," or life force, flow.

Over the ages, cupping therapy expanded throughout various nations and areas, adjusting to the customs and beliefs of the local medical community. During the Islamic Golden Era, cupping techniques underwent tremendous refinement thanks in large part to the contributions of Islamic scholars.

Globalization has led to a rise in the use of cupping in alternative medicine, fusing traditional wisdom with cutting-edge techniques.

DIFFERENT CUPPING METHODS

A range of treatments are included in cupping therapy, each with its advantages and method of operation. The most prevalent types consist of:

1. Dry cupping: In this technique, cups are placed on particular body spots without any oil or cream preparation beforehand. By drawing the skin and underlying tissues upward and creating a vacuum, the cups help to improve blood circulation and relieve tense muscles.

2. Wet Cupping (Hijama): Following dry cupping, practitioners use this technique to make tiny skin incisions to extract a tiny amount of blood. Toxins are said to be eliminated, and general well-being is enhanced.

3. A classic method called "Fire Cupping" involves the practitioner creating a vacuum inside the cup using a flame before applying it to the patient's skin. The cups are left in position for a predetermined amount of time after the flame is extinguished, causing suction.

4. Massage Cupping: After applying oil or cream, cups are moved over the skin's surface to create a massage-like sensation. This method is frequently applied to relieve tense muscles and encourage relaxation.

Based on the principles of traditional medicine, each treatment seeks to balance the body's energy flow, relieve pain, and increase blood flow.

ADVANTAGES AND DANGERS

It is thought that cupping therapy provides several health advantages, such as increased circulation, pain reduction, and muscle relaxation. Back pain, migraines, respiratory problems, and stress are among the diseases that it is frequently used to treat. It is believed that the suction produced by the cups will improve blood flow, which could speed up the healing process for damaged tissues.

Like any treatment technique, cupping has hazards associated with it. At the cupping areas, some people may have transient bruises, skin irritations, or discomforts. The degree of cupping can be changed according to each person's tolerance and medical circumstances. Before receiving cupping therapy, anyone who is pregnant, has specific skin disorders or is prone to bleeding should speak with a healthcare provider.

HOW THE BODY REACTS TO CUPPING

There are several different mechanisms underlying cupping therapy. It is believed that the suction produced by the cups lifts the skin and underlying tissues, boosting lymphatic fluid flow and blood circulation. It is thought that this improved circulation helps the body get rid of waste materials and poisons while giving cells the oxygen and nutrition they need.

According to traditional Chinese medical theory, cupping is also thought to affect the body's energy meridians. Practitioners seek to cure both physical and energetic imbalances by restoring equilibrium inside the body by harmonizing the flow of qi.

Moreover, it is thought that the negative pressure produced by cupping releases tension in the muscles and initiates the relaxation response. In addition to enhancing joint mobility and reducing pain, this can also increase general well-being.

Cupping treatment employs a variety of procedures to address a wide range of health conditions by balancing energy flow, improving circulation, and eliciting a therapeutic response in the body. It blends traditional wisdom with modern applications. Before adding cupping to one's wellness regimen, it is imperative to speak with a licensed healthcare provider, just like with any alternative therapy.

CHAPTER FOUR

THE SCIENTIFIC BASIS OF CELLULITE CUPPING

THE WORKINGS OF CUPPING TO TREAT CELLULITE

Since it has been used for millennia in traditional medicine, cupping treatment has drawn interest due to its potential for treating cellulite. There are several different ways that cupping reduces cellulite. The enhancement of blood circulation is one important factor. The cups' suction increases blood flow to the targeted locations, improving the supply of nutrients and oxygen. It is thought that this improved circulation will speed up the breakdown of toxins and fat deposits that cause cellulite to form.

Cupping is also believed to activate the lymphatic system. The cups' suction and negative pressure may aid in removing waste products and extra fluid from the tissues, which would lessen edema and the cellulite-related dimpled look. Cupping may also facilitate the loosening of fascial limitations. The cups' mild pulling action on the skin and underlying tissues may aid in the connective tissue's stretching and loosening, which could assist in reducing the appearance of cellulite.

INVESTIGATIONS AND RESULTS

Although there has been some research on cupping therapy for cellulite, more thorough investigations are required as the field of scientific investigation into this treatment is still in its infancy. Although preliminary research has indicated some advantages, the quality of the data differs.

According to a 2018 study that was published in the Journal of Acupuncture and Meridian Studies, cupping therapy dramatically improved the texture and look of cellulite-affected women's skin. Nevertheless, the sample size was small, and bigger cohorts would need to be studied to confirm these results.

Another investigation into the effects of cupping on subcutaneous fat layers was published in the Journal of Alternative and Complementary Medicine in 2017. The outcomes showed a decrease in the circumference of the thighs and an improvement in the cellulite's look. However, the study's shortcomings—such as its brief duration and limited sample size—highlight the need for more thorough examinations.

EXPERT VIEWS ON CUPPING TO REDUCE CELLULITE

Experts differ in their opinions about how effective cupping is at reducing cellulite. Proponents of alternative therapies and certain practitioners argue that cupping can be a useful addition to a comprehensive cellulite treatment plan, highlighting its potential to improve tissue elasticity, lymphatic drainage, and blood circulation.

Skeptics in the medical world, however, point out that there isn't enough solid scientific data to support cupping as a treatment for cellulite and advise against depending on it alone. They contend that additional studies are required to determine the efficacy of cupping and comprehend its long-term effects.

More well-planned, large-scale studies are needed to definitively confirm the efficacy of cupping for cellulite removal, even though there is preliminary research and anecdotal evidence to support its potential advantages. Individual results may differ, as with many alternative therapies, thus speaking with medical professionals is advised before including cupping in a cellulite treatment strategy.

CHAPTER FIVE

TYPES OF CELLULITE CUPPING TECHNIQUES

WITHOUT WET CUPPING

Using cups on the skin to produce a vacuum seal that encourages blood flow and releases tense muscles is known as "dry cupping," a traditional therapy method. Dry cupping is thought to encourage lymphatic drainage and circulation in the context of cellulite treatment, which may help lessen the appearance of cellulite. The cups produce a vacuum that draws blood to the skin's surface, facilitating the delivery of nutrients and oxygen to the desired locations.

MOIST CUPPING

Wet Cupping, also referred to as "hijama," is a more intrusive type of cupping in which tiny skin incisions are made before the cups are applied. A tiny amount of blood is drawn out of the body along with toxins and other impurities by the suction that the cups create. Although wet cupping is not a popular method of treating cellulite, some advocates claim that it can help break up stagnant fluids and enhance circulation in general, which may help reduce cellulite.

CUPPING MASSAGE

Traditional cupping is combined with massage techniques to create Massage Cupping. Using lubricants on the skin, practitioners glide the cups over the body to produce a light massage. This technique is supposed to promote lymphatic drainage, increase blood flow, and dissolve fascial adhesions. Massage cupping attempts to improve the suppleness of connective tissues about cellulite, which may lessen the skin's dimpled look.

RAPID CUPPING

The technique known as "flash cupping" involves applying and removing cups very quickly. It is thought that by stimulating the skin and underlying tissues, this technique will encourage lymphatic drainage and a flushing effect. While there isn't much scientific proof to back up its effectiveness in reducing cellulite, some practitioners use flash cupping to energize the regions that are being treated.

SILICONE ENCASEMENT

Using silicone cups in place of conventional glass or plastic cups is known as silicone cupping. Because silicone cups are flexible, applying suction may be done more precisely and with greater care. Silicone cupping is a cellulite therapy that is said to increase blood flow, break down fatty deposits, and stimulate the creation of collagen. Silicone cups are particularly ideal for usage on curved or delicate body parts because of their flexibility.

There are a variety of cupping treatments for cellulite, each with its own specialization and set of claimed advantages.

While cupping may help some people with their cellulite symptoms, it's important to remember that there is little scientific evidence to support its efficacy and that each person will react differently. To be sure cupping therapy is safe and suitable for their particular condition, people should speak with medical professionals before beginning treatment.

CHAPTER SIX

SELECTING THE APPROPRIATE TOOLS AND CUPS

TYPES & MATERIALS OF CUPS

Selecting the right materials and cup types is essential to providing a comfortable and successful cupping therapy session. Glass, plastic, silicone, and bamboo are among the materials that are frequently used to make cups. Because they are transparent and enable therapists to observe the patient's skin while receiving therapy, glass cups are conventional and frequently chosen. Conversely, silicone cups are pliable and simple to squeeze, which makes them appropriate for dynamic cupping methods.

There are different types of cups; some are meant to be placed immobile, while others are meant to move dynamically throughout the body. Static cupping is a technique in which stationary cups are positioned on particular acupuncture sites and held there for a predetermined amount of time. Dynamic cups—such as those equipped with pumps or suction bulbs—are used in massage treatments that include moving the cups around the body to simulate a massage. The therapy objectives and the preferences of the patient and the treating professional will determine which of these approaches is best.

CHOOSING THE RIGHT TOOLS FOR THE RIGHT BODY PARTS'

The human body is made up of many areas with different anatomical features and sensitivities. As a result, choosing the right cupping instruments for the various body parts is crucial to guaranteeing a secure and efficient procedure. Practitioners frequently choose larger cups for larger muscle groups and wider areas because they may cover a greater surface area and provide effective suction and therapeutic results. Conversely, smaller cups are appropriate for portions of the body that are more fragile or have complex anatomical features.

For example, smaller and softer cups are needed for facial cupping to fit the delicate facial skin. greater cups with powerful suction may be better for treating the shoulders and back since they can efficiently target greater muscle groups. Additionally, because silicone cups are more flexible and adaptable to the body's contours, practitioners may decide to use them for joints and bony areas.

SAFETY MEASURES

Although cupping therapy has several health advantages, patient safety must always come first throughout treatment. To avoid any negative consequences or injuries, practitioners need to be well-versed in safety measures.

First and foremost, the length of time cups are left on the skin must be taken into account, as doing so might cause irritation or bruises. It's critical to keep an eye on the skin's reaction and modify the treatment as necessary.

Additionally, practitioners need to use caution while applying suction because too much pressure can hurt or harm the skin. To prevent illnesses, it is essential to practice good hygiene. Disposable cups or thoroughly sterilized reusable cups in between sessions should be used. To protect their safety and well-being, clients with certain medical conditions, such as skin disorders or problems with blood clotting, should be properly evaluated before receiving cupping therapy.

Choosing cups and other equipment for cupping therapy is a sophisticated procedure that calls for careful thought out of factors including safety measures, styles, and materials. Practitioners can increase the efficacy of cupping treatments while maintaining the safety of their customers by being aware of the various needs of various body parts and giving priority to safety precautions.

CHAPTER SEVEN

GETTING READY FOR A SESSION OF CUPPING

CONSULTATION AND EVALUATION

A successful session in the field of cupping therapy begins with a comprehensive consultation and assessment. Practitioners have a thorough conversation with the client to learn about their medical history, present state of health, and specific issues before starting any kind of treatment. This consultation is essential because it enables the practitioner to customize the cupping procedure to the specific requirements of the patient. It contains questions regarding current medical issues, prescription drugs, and any ailments that should not be used in conjunction with cupping therapy.

In addition, a practical evaluation could be carried out to pinpoint particular points of strain, discomfort, or unbalance.

Through this physical assessment, the practitioner can precisely arrange cups for the best effect and gauge the right amount of suction for the best outcomes. Using the consultation and assessment procedure, professionals can devise a customized and focused strategy, augmenting the comprehensive efficacy of the cupping session.

SANITATION AND HYGIENE

To protect the client's safety and well-being as well as the practitioner's, cupping therapy requires strict adherence to high standards of hygiene and sanitation. Practitioners are required to thoroughly clean and sterilize all cupping equipment, including cups, pumps, and any additional attachments, before each session. Sometimes it's better to use disposable cups to reduce the possibility of cross-contamination. Following stringent hygienic procedures is crucial, including sanitizing hands both before and after the treatment and wearing disposable gloves.

Additionally, to avoid any possible illnesses, practitioners need to teach their customers the value of maintaining good personal cleanliness. A favorable experience is enhanced by hygienic and cozy surroundings, which build confidence in the therapeutic process. Cupping practitioners show their dedication to providing a secure and hygienic environment for patients seeking this alternative therapy by maintaining strict hygiene and sanitation standards.

MENTALLY GETTING THE CLIENT READY

An essential component of a good cupping session is the client's mental preparation. Applying suction cups to the skin is known as "cupping marks" or "she," and it might result in markings due to the expulsion of toxins and stagnant blood. Providing the client with information on these marks, their transient nature, and the therapeutic advantages of the procedure aids in controlling expectations and allaying worries.

Practitioners should advise customers on mental and relaxation strategies in addition to outlining the physical components. A more peaceful and tranquil atmosphere, enhanced by soft lighting and soothing music, might help patients feel better mentally. To foster mindfulness and facilitate the release of tension, practitioners may also advise clients to concentrate on their breathing.

The client's mental readiness is essential to guaranteeing a successful and positive cupping session. Practitioners can improve a client's comfort level and receptiveness to the therapy process by addressing any concerns or uncertainties, which can lead to a more effective and fulfilling outcome.

CHAPTER EIGHT

CARRYING OUT CELLULITE CUPPING THERAPY

A STEP-BY-STEP GUIDE TO A CUPPING SESSION

A detailed protocol must be followed when implementing cupping therapy for cellulite to guarantee a thorough and productive session. First and foremost, it's imperative to start with a comprehensive evaluation of the client's cellulite areas. This assessment aids in pinpointing the precise areas that need care and cupping therapy method customization.

Start the session by smearing the targeted cellulite areas with an appropriate lubricant or oil. This makes it easier for the cups to glide over the skin and keeps the therapy session pain-free. Selecting a lubricant that matches the skin type and improves the cups' glide without sacrificing their suction power is crucial.

Specialized cups are placed on the skin's surface to begin the real cupping procedure. When these cups are applied, a vacuum is created that lifts the skin and produces a suction effect. Selecting the appropriate cup type is crucial for treating cellulite, taking into account elements like dimensions, composition, and design. Silicone cups are a popular choice for cupping cellulite because of their flexibility and mild yet powerful suction.

Therapists must carefully move the cups over the cellulite-prone areas throughout the cupping therapy. Use a method that combines gliding and stationary movements to reduce cellulite as much as possible. By treating the underlying causes of cellulite formation, the suction action helps to increase blood circulation, lymphatic drainage, and collagen creation.

When concentrating on particular cellulite locations, pay attention to the uneven texture and distinctive dimpled look. Make sure you thoroughly cover the afflicted areas by moving the cups in zigzag or circular patterns. Depending on the client's comfort level and the degree of cellulite, modify the pressure and duration. Throughout the session, it's critical to stay in touch with the client to check on their well-being and address any issues.

CHANGING THE INTENSITY OF CUPPING

A crucial part of customizing the therapy to each patient's needs is varying the strength of the cupping process. The cups' suction strength can be adjusted to change the intensity. It may be beneficial for novices or those with sensitive skin to begin with lower suction settings and increase them gradually as tolerance develops. On the other hand, people who are used to cupping therapy could choose to target deep-seated cellulite with a stronger suction.

Post-cupping care is essential to maximize therapeutic efficacy and reduce adverse effects. Encourage customers to drink plenty of water, refrain from exerting themselves right after the session, and moisturize the regions that were treated regularly. Inform them of the anticipated results and the necessity of several sessions for the best possible cellulite removal.

Applying cupping therapy for cellulite requires a methodical, step-by-step process that targets particular areas with varied cupping intensities. This meticulous procedure guarantees a safe and personalized experience for the individuals seeking this alternative therapy in addition to addressing cellulite concerns.

CHAPTER NINE

AFTER-CUPPING MANAGEMENT AND SUGGESTIONS

INSTRUCTIONS FOR AFTERCARE

Prioritising aftercare is essential to maximizing benefits and minimizing potential negative effects following a cupping therapy session. The first piece of advice is to drink lots of water to stay hydrated. Enhancing the body's natural detoxification processes, drinking enough water aids in the removal of toxins generated during cupping. Moreover, the cleansing effects of quitting alcohol and coffee a few hours after starting a cup can be increased.

It's also recommended to move gently and stretch lightly following cupping therapy. This increases circulation and lessens stiffness, which improves the treatment's overall efficacy. However, it is best to avoid hard exercise and demanding activities right after cupping to give the body time to heal and avoid putting additional tension on the areas that were treated.

Because of the effect of the suction on blood vessels, skin darkening or bruises are frequently experienced following cupping. To lessen bruising and ease any discomfort, use an arnica cream or soothing ointment for the affected regions. Clothing that fits comfortably and loosely might also help to avoid skin irritation.

POSSIBLE SIDE EFFECTS AND HOW TO HANDLE THEM

Although cupping therapy is thought to be safe, there could be some unintended consequences that you should be aware of. Common side effects include bruises, discolorations, and mild soreness, which go away in a few days. However, it is best to speak with a healthcare provider if the bruises are serious or if there are a lot of them.

There are rare instances where people may feel lightheaded or dizzy following cupping. After a session, this can be controlled by resting for a few minutes and then gradually sitting up. It is important to visit a doctor if symptoms worsen.

Cupping occasionally results in blisters or transient skin discomfort. Infection can be avoided by cleaning the region and using an antibacterial ointment. To prevent making the situation worse, it's crucial to refrain from picking or scratching at any blisters.

RECURRING MEETINGS AND UPKEEP

The number of cupping sessions is determined by the particular ailment being treated as well as the goals of each individual. Some people might get by with just one session, but others who have ongoing problems might need to come in for regular check-ups. To find the ideal frequency of cupping treatments, consult with a certified practitioner about a customized treatment plan.

Maintaining your health and well-being over time may benefit from routine maintenance sessions.

These sessions can support any new problems that may arise, keep the benefits of cupping going, and stop symptoms from returning. Treatment plans can be modified in response to each patient's unique reaction and changing health demands when there is open communication between the patient and the cupping therapist.

A comprehensive and successful cupping therapy experience is facilitated by appropriate aftercare, knowledge of possible adverse effects, and a customized follow-up strategy. People can maximize the advantages of cupping while guaranteeing a secure and comfortable healing process by combining these components.

CHAPTER TEN

INTEGRATING CUPPING WITH ADDITIONAL THERAPIES

NUTRITION AND DIET

Cupping therapy along with other complementary methods can provide a comprehensive approach to general health. Diet and nutrition are important factors to take into account. Having a healthy, well-balanced diet is essential for promoting the body's natural healing processes.

Cupping therapy can work in concert with a healthy diet high in antioxidants, vitamins, and minerals because of its capacity to improve blood circulation and encourage detoxification. Together, they may strengthen the body's ability to flush out toxins and promote tissue healing, building a stronger base for overall health.

PHYSICAL ACTIVITY AND EXERCISE

The advantages of cupping therapy can be increased by integrating it into an active lifestyle that involves frequent exercise and physical activity. Increased muscle flexibility, blood circulation, and general vitality are all benefits of exercise. Together with cupping, which helps release tension in the muscles and encourages relaxation, the combination can be especially beneficial for treating musculoskeletal problems. This mixture may lessen the chance of damage, hasten the body's recuperation from physical activity, and increase the overall effectiveness of physiological processes.

SKINCARE PROTOCOLS

Cupping therapy can be easily used with skincare routines to improve skin health. Cupping is well-recognised to increase the formation of collagen, enhance blood circulation to the skin, and facilitate lymphatic fluid evacuation.

Cupping treatment may help to improve skin elasticity, minimize the appearance of fine lines, and provide the appearance of a more radiant complexion when combined with a customized skincare program that includes hydrating products. This all-encompassing strategy promotes the interior and exterior facets of healthy skin.

EXTRA TREATMENTS FOR BETTER OUTCOMES

Combining cupping with other therapy techniques can be beneficial to promote overall well-being. In addition to cupping, modalities including massage, acupuncture, and aromatherapy can help with specific health issues and encourage relaxation. Combining cupping with acupuncture, for example, can improve the overall efficacy of both treatments since they complement each other in balancing the body's energy flow and promoting the body's natural healing processes. Comparably, adding cupping to a massage treatment can offer a multifaceted strategy for relieving tense muscles and encouraging calm.

Additionally, cupping therapy can be combined with mindfulness exercises like yoga or meditation to enhance mental and emotional well-being. The benefits of cupping for stress relief and relaxation are consistent with the objectives of mindfulness practices, resulting in a more harmonious relationship between the mind and body.

A comprehensive and synergistic approach to health and well-being can be created by integrating cupping therapy with different lifestyle factors and additional therapeutic approaches. The integration of many factors, such as dietary optimization, active lifestyle adoption, skincare, and other therapeutic modalities, can enhance the advantages of cupping and promote a more comprehensive and well-rounded approach to overall well-being.

CHAPTER ELEVEN

TYPICAL PROBLEMS AND THEIR FIXES

RESOLVING PAIN OR UNEASE

In many professions, including therapy, fitness, and healthcare, one of the most frequent challenges is helping people with their pain or discomfort. Professionals must handle situations involving clients or patients who are in pain during a session with compassion and understanding. First and first, it's critical to have an open line of communication with the person, encouraging them to describe the source of their discomfort and express it. This makes it possible for practitioners to fully comprehend the problem and adjust their strategy accordingly.

When a client might expect pain or discomfort during a procedure, specialists should inform them in advance. Managing expectations can be achieved by reassuring them of the transient nature of the discomfort and giving clear information about the possible feelings.

Incorporating relaxation methods during the session, like guided imagery or deep breathing, can also help to reduce physical discomfort and foster a more enjoyable experience.

HANDLING BRUISING

Whether it comes from massage therapy, physical training, or medical procedures, bruising can be an unanticipated and unsettling consequence of many different disciplines. Practitioners must take a proactive and open approach to treating bruises. To reduce the chance of bruising, one important tactic is to evaluate and modify the pressure or intensity used during the session. A good warm-up, appropriate technique, and frequent client discussions about their comfort level are all essential to avoiding bruises.

When bruising does happen, professionals should be the first to recognize the problem and show compassion. Educating people about the typical length of time and the natural healing process of bruises helps allay fears. To hasten the healing process, practitioners can also suggest topical or home medicines. Building a connection of empathy and support with customers during these kinds of situations is essential to preserving their trust and guaranteeing their continued involvement.

OVERCOMING CLIENT OPPOSITION

When offering novel and unfamiliar concepts or practices, professionals frequently run across client opposition. Establishing a cooperative and communicative atmosphere is crucial for overcoming resistance. It is important for professionals to actively listen to their clients' worries and anxieties while respecting their viewpoints. By allowing clients to participate in the decision-making process, professionals can empower people and increase their openness to suggested changes.

The key to overcoming opposition is education. Giving clients thorough and lucid explanations of the advantages and reasoning behind a specific strategy will help them understand the process. Professionals should also stress that the adjustments are flexible and progressive, allowing clients to adjust at their speed. Establishing a trustworthy relationship that makes customers feel understood and encouraged is essential to overcoming resistance and fostering positive results.

TROUBLESHOOTING COMMON ISSUES

To guarantee the seamless provision of services, troubleshooting common issues is an ongoing effort in any professional practice. Promptly recognizing and resolving issues can improve the overall customer experience. Creating frequent feedback loops and encouraging clients to share any issues or challenges they may be having is one successful tactic.

By being proactive, practitioners may address problems immediately and make the necessary changes to increase customer satisfaction.

Practitioners should look at the underlying causes of frequent problems rather than only treating the symptoms. Professionals can apply focused solutions by comprehending the fundamental causes of problems. Working together to solve problems with clients creates a sense of cooperation that increases the likelihood that clients will participate in problem-solving. Maintaining up-to-date knowledge of industry developments and engaging in ongoing professional development are other factors that support proactive troubleshooting, giving practitioners the tools they need to overcome obstacles.